Legal & Disclaimer

The information contained in this book is not designed to replace or take the place of any form of medication or professional medical advice. The information in this book has been provided for educational and entertainment purposes only.

The information contained in this book has been compiled from sources deemed reliable, and it is accurate to the best of the Author's knowledge. However, the Author cannot guarantee its accuracy and validity so cannot be held liable for any errors or omissions. Changes are periodically made to this book. You must consult your doctor or get professional medical advice before using any of the suggested remedies, techniques, or information in this book.

Upon using the information contained in this book, you agree to hold harmless the Author from and against any damages, costs and expenses, including any legal fees, potentially resulting from the application of any of the information provided by this guide. This disclaimer applies to any damages or injury caused by the use and application, whether directly or indirectly, of any advice or information presented, whether for breach of contract, tort, negligence, personal injury, criminal intent, or under any other cause of action.

You agree to accept all the risks of using the information presented inside this book. You need to consult a professional medical practitioner in order to ensure you are both able & healthy enough to participate in this program.

Contents

Introduction

There are countless diets out there that argue to be the best for you. But there is one thing that all these diets agree on – the emphasis and consumption of fresh, whole ingredients while minimizing processed foods. Health and wellness experts agree that these kinds of food can pave the way to a holistic well-being.

What is Wholefoods Plant-based Diet?

Simply put, the whole-food plant-based diet focuses on minimally processed foods, focusing on plants. It limits or avoids consumption of meat altogether, and excludes refined foods such as added sugar, processed oils and white flour from your diet. It also promotes local and organically grown produce, which includes vegetables, fruits, whole grains, legumes, seeds, ad nuts.

Benefits of Wholefoods Plant-based Diet

Making the dietary choices with this diet can result to a host of beneficial results. For example, the whole-foods plant-based diet helps facilitate weight loss, due to the high-fiber content of the nature of foods eaten. Along with this, the exclusion of processed foods makes a more winning combination.

Apart from benefiting your waistline, it can also help lower your risk and reduce symptoms of certain chronic diseases such as heart disease, cancer, and diabetes. Cognitive health can also benefit from this, as plant compounds and anti-oxidants from plant sources show that these help in slowing or preventing cognitive decline and the progression of Alzheimer's disease.

People who follow this diet tend to have smaller environmental footprints. By adopting sustainable eating habits, one can reduce gas emissions, water consumption, and land used for factory farming – all of which are factors in global warming and environmental degradation.

Lunch And Dinner Recipes

Soups And Stews

Minestrone Soup

Servings: 2

Prep Time: 5 minutes   Cook Time: 20 minutes

Ingredients:

1 large onion, chopped

2 medium carrots, chopped

1 stalk celery, chopped

2 large cloves garlic, minced

1 can (14.5 ounces) diced tomatoes, undrained

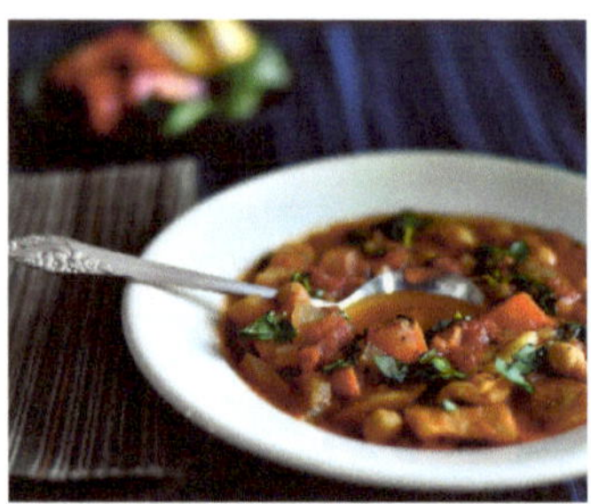

1 can (15.5 ounces) cannellini beans, or other white beans, drained and rinsed

1 medium zucchini, diced

4 cups vegetable broth

1 tsp dried basil

½ tsp dried oregano

salt and ground black pepper

Procedure:

1. Over medium fire, heat a large saucepan. Place onions, carrots, celery, and garlic into the pan and cook until softened.

2. Add 1-2 tablespoons of water at a time as needed.

3. Stir in the tomatoes with their juices, beans, zucchini, and broth.

4. Add in basil, oregano, and sprinkle with salt and pepper to taste.

5. Bring mixture to a boil, reduce heat to low, and continue to simmer until vegetables are tender.

6. Serve hot.

Pesto Soup with Asparagus, Zucchini, and Peas

Servings: 4

Prep Time: 10 minutes   Cook Time: 20 minutes

Ingredients:

1 bunch asparagus, chopped

1 cup English peas

3 medium-sized zucchini, sliced

1 medium onion, chopped

2 cloves garlic, chopped

118 ml vegetable broth

1 can light coconut milk

½ lemon, juiced

1 tsp salt

¼ tsp pepper

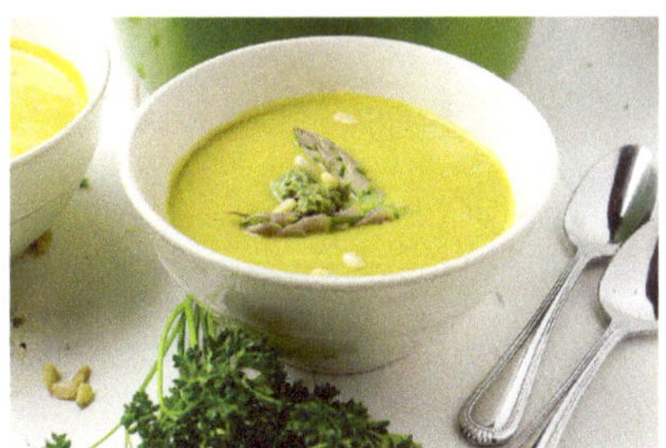

Pesto:

354g basil leaves, tightly packed

1/2 cup parsley, tightly packed

3 cloves garlic

1 tbsp light miso, white or red

3 tbsp nutritional yeast

30 g pine nuts

3 tbsp lemon juice

Salt and pepper to taste

Procedure:

1.   Blend all ingredients of pesto in a food processor until smooth. Set aside.

2. In a large soup pot over medium heat, saute onion and garlic in ¼ cup water until fragrant.

3. Chop off the rough ends of the asparagus, then cut into 1 inch pieces. Add to the pot with the zucchini, peas, vegetable broth and coconut milk.

4. Cover and simmer for 20 minutes, or until asparagus is tender.

5. Once the asparagus is tender, add in the lemon juice, salt, and pepper. Blend in a high-speed blender in batches until creamy.

6. Transfer back to the soup pot until ready to serve.

7. Ladle into soup bowls and garnish with a dollop of pesto.

Black Bean Soup with Sweet Potatoes

Servings: 5

Prep Time: 10 minutes   Cook Time: 20 minutes

Ingredients:

¼ cup water or vegetable broth for sauteing

3 cups fresh black beans, picked over and rinsed

1 large onion, diced

1 large sweet potato, peeled and cubed

1 large red pepper, seeded and diced

2 ribs celery, diced

4 cups vegetable broth

2 cups water

1 tsp ground cumin

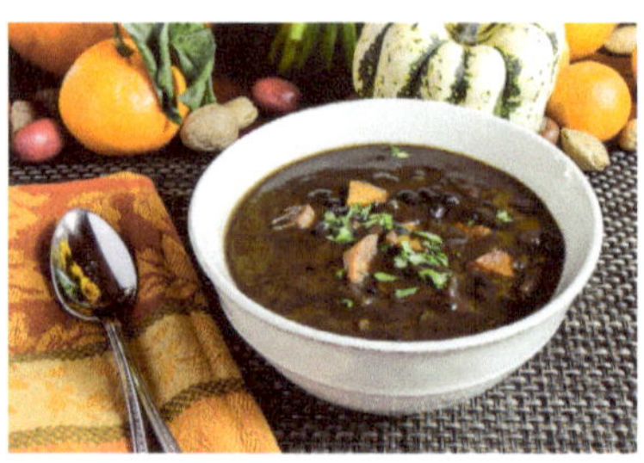

½ tsp ground coriander

½ tsp salt or to taste

1/3 tsp ground pepper

1 large avocado, diced

1 tbsp cilantro, minced

80 ml vegan sour cream

Procedure:

1. In a large pot over medium heat, saute the onion, celery, sweet potato and bell pepper in ¼ cup water or vegetable broth until soft and translucent.

2. Add 3 cups of homemade black beans, 2 cups water, and 4 cups vegetable broth.

3. Add cumin, coriander, salt, and pepper.

4. Simmer on medium until the vegetables and sweet potatoes are soft, about 20 minutes.

5. Once slightly cooled, transfer half of the soup into a blender until smooth. Pour back into the pot and mix well.

6. Serve topped with diced avocado and a sprinkling of minced cilantro.

7. Add a dollop of vegan sour cream.

Mushroom Quinoa Soup

Servings: 4

Prep Time: 10 minutes   Cook Time: 20 minutes

Ingredients:

¼ cup water

½ yellow onion, chopped

2 cloves garlic, minced

227g mushrooms, sliced

1 small zucchini cut in half lengthwise, then sliced

120g uncooked quinoa

4 cups vegetable broth

1 tsp oregano

½ tsp thyme

2 tbsp flour

1 cup unsweetened non-dairy milk

½ tsp salt

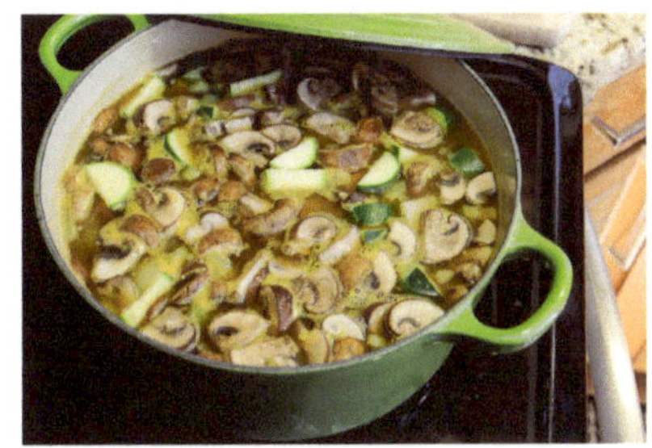

Pepper to taste

Procedure:

1. Saute onions in about ¼ cup water until translucent.

2. Add garlic and mushrooms and continue to saute until mushrooms start to soften and wilt.

3. Add zucchini, quinoa, and vegetable broth. Continue cooking until mushrooms are done.

4. In a small bowl, mix ½ cup of the non-dairy milk with 2 tbsp flour until smooth. Add this to the mushroom mixture along with the other ½ cup milk.

5. Stir to combine and heat until creamy and thickened.

6. Add salt and pepper to taste.

Curry Corn Soup

Servings: 4

Prep Time: 10 minutes   Cook Time: 15 minutes

Ingredients:

½ onion, chopped

3 shallots, chopped

2 cloves garlic, minced

½ green pepper, diced

2 carrots, diced

6 red potatoes, diced

1 can organic corn

1 tsp curry powder

½ ginger powder, or more to taste

½ tsp coriander, or more to taste

½ tsp turmeric

1 can coconut milk

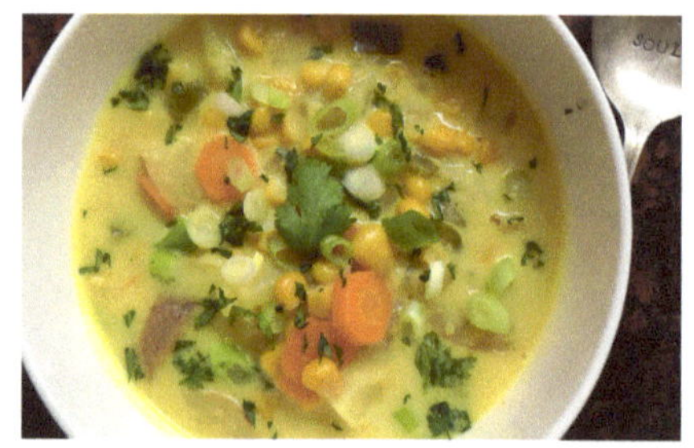

1 cup water

Juice of 1 lime

Salt, a pinch to taste

Splash of tamari or coconut aminos to taste

Cilantro and Scallions for garnish

Procedure:

1. In a soup pot, saute carrots and shallots in oil. Add the garlic and continue to saute until soft.

2. Add the green pepper, carrots, and potatoes.

3. Add in the coriander, turmeric, curry powder, and canned corn. Toss around to coat the vegetables.

4. Add the coconut milk, water, lime juice, a pinch of salt, and a splash of tamari or coconut aminos.

5. Cover and cook until potatoes are soft.

6. Taste and adjust salt.

7. Serve with fresh cilantro and scallions on top.

Lentil Kale Soup

Servings: 5

Prep Time: 10 minutes   Cook Time: 20 minutes

Ingredients:

473g cooked brown lentils or 1 cup uncooked

½ large onion, chopped

3 cloves garlic, peeled and minced

3 medium carrots, peeled and chopped

2 stalks celery, chopped

4 cups vegetable broth

2 cups water

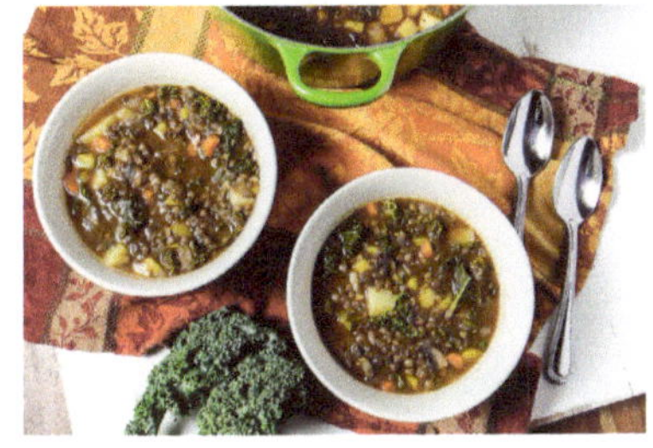

3 ounces tomato paste

½ tsp coriander

½ tsp cumin

½ tsp salt or to taste

¼ tsp freshly ground pepper

1 large potato, peeled and chopped

2-3 large leaves kale, stems removed and roughly chopped

Procedure:

1. Add ¼ cup veggie broth to a large pot and saute the onion, carrot, celery, and garlic for several minutes until soft and tender.

2. Add more broth along with the tomato paste.

3. Add the rest of the ingredients except for kale, and stir to combine.

4. If using uncooked lentils, rinse and pick over and add them to the pot along with 2 extra cups of water.

5. Cook on medium for about 15 - 20 minutes.

6. Add the kale, stir, and cook until lentils are ready.

7. Serve hot.

Cold Cucumber Soup

Servings: 6

Prep Time: 15 minutes

Ingredients:

800g cucumbers, peeled, seeded, and cut into 3-inch pieces

¼ red onion, roughly chopped

1 clove garlic, skinned

8 large mint leaves

1 tsp maple syrup

2 tbsp lemon juice

170g plain homemade or store-bought soy yogurt

½ cup water or more

1 avocado, chopped

Salt to taste

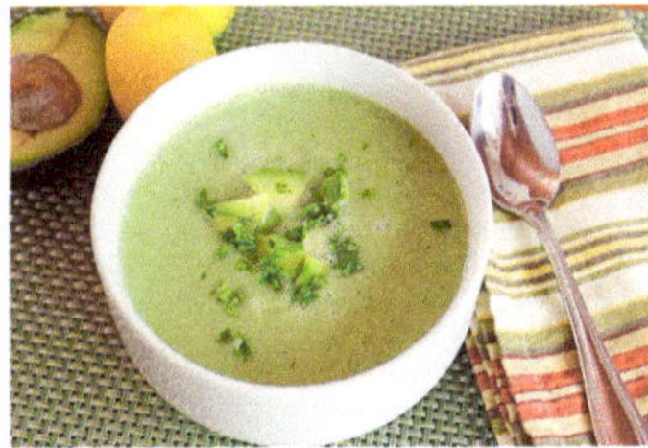

Procedure:

1. Place all the ingredients except the avocado in a Vitamix or food processor with ½ cup of water.

2. Pulse a few times so the ingredients are coarsely chopped, then process until smooth.

3. Thin with more water if needed.

4. Transfer to a bowl and refrigerate 2 hours to overnight, until well chilled.

5. Ladle soup into bowls and top with avocado slices.

Salads

Morrocan Salad Bowl

Servings: 2

Prep Time: 15 minutes   Cook Time: 15 minutes

Ingredients:

½ cup uncooked couscous or quinoa

¼ cup water to cook couscous or quinoa

½ cup cooked chickpeas

20 cherry tomatoes, quartered

1 medium cucumber, diced

1 small courgette, sliced thickly

1 small aubergine, sliced thickly

15 black olives

Handful of fresh mint, chopped thinly

¼ pomegranate, seeds only

2 garlic cloves, finely chopped

Salt and pepper

3 tbsp olive oil

½ tsp chili

1 tsp cumin

1 tsp sweet paprika

A few slices of preserved lemons, store-bought or as per recipe below

Quick Preserved Lemons (to make at least a day ahead):

3 small unwaxed lemons

45 ml lemon juice

1 garlic clove, crushed with the edge of a knife

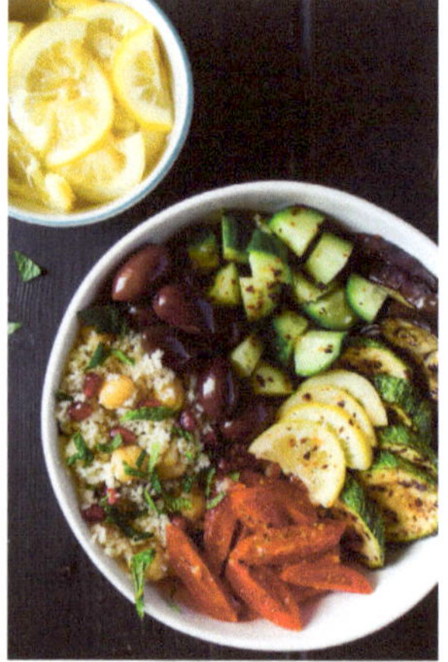

½ chili, chopped

2 tsp sea salt

35 gm sugar

Procedure:

1. In a pot or kettle, boil ¼ cup water. Once boiling, pour over couscous and immediately cover with a lid. If using quinoa, cook according to package directions.

2. In a small pan, heat 2 tbsp of olive oil. Saute garlic until soft and fragrant.

3. Add in tomatoes and season with salt and pepper. Saute until juices start to come out.

4. Brush aubergine and courgette slices with a little bit of oil and grill over a griddle until cooked on both sides. Sprinkle with salt, cumin, paprika, and touch of chili afterwards.

5. Fluff up cooked couscous with a fork, mix it with chickpeas, pomegranate seeds, and freshly cut mint.

6. Divide olives, grilled veggies, raw cucumber, couscous, and sauteed tomatoes between 2 bowls.

7. Use garlicky oil and tomatoes as a dressing. (from step 3)

8. Serve with a few slices of finely chopped lemon.

To make the preserved lemons:

1. Scrub lemons very well. If they have a wax coating, immerse them in boiling water for a few minutes to dissolve it.

2. Cut them into half lengthwise and then into very thin slices, as thin as you can.

3. Pound 1 tsp of salt and chili in a mortar and pestle until you get a thick paste.

4. Place chili paste, the rest of the salt, sugar, and lemon juice in a bowl. Add lemon slices and rub the salt-sugar mixture into them.

5. Stick crushed garlic into the mixture. Cover and refrigerate at least 1 day prior to using.

Roasted Vegetable Salad with Avocado Dressing

Servings: 2

Prep Time: 5 minutes   Cook Time: 20 minutes

Ingredients:

Roasted vegetables:

2 small potatoes, cubed

1 medium sweet potato, cubed

1 red bell pepper, chopped

1 cup baby brussel sprouts, halved

3 tbsp olive oil

1 tbsp dried oregano

Salt and black pepper to taste

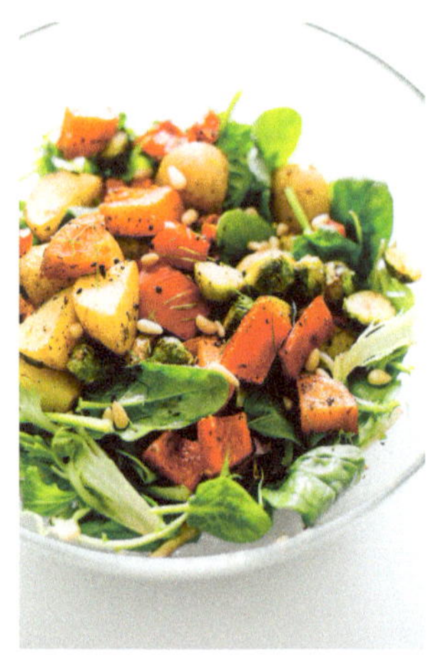

Greens:

1 bag mixed salad greens

1 tbsp red wine vinegar

1 tbsp olive oil

¼ cup pine nuts

Salt and pepper

Avocado Dressing:

½ avocado

3 tbsp olive oil

2 tsp rice vinegar

1 clove garlic

5 tbsp coconut water

Salt and pepper to taste

Procedure:

1. Preheat oven to 180C. Place vegetables on a lined baking sheet and roast until caramelized, about 20 minutes.

2. In a mixing bowl, add chopped red bell pepper and halved baby brussel sprouts to, along with olive oil, dried oregano, and salt and pepper. Toss to combine.

3. Mix together the salad greens, with red wine vinegar, olive oil, pine nuts, salt and pepper in a salad bowl. Toss to combine.

4. To make the dressing, combine avocado, olive oil, rice vinegar, garlic, coconut water, salt, and pepper into a blender. Blend until smooth. If dressing is a little thick, add a little more coconut water and blend.

5. Add in the roasted veggies and toss well to combine. Serve.

Tomatoes, Chickpea, and Spinach Salad

Servings: 2

Prep Time: 10 minutes   Cook Time: 10 minutes

Ingredients:

400gm cooked chickpeas

1 cup baby spinach, rinsed

5 spring onions, chopped

5 tomatoes, medium, chopped

1 red pepper, chopped

⅓ cup parsley, chopped

1 tbsp balsamic vinegar

Juice of ½ lemon

2 tbsp olive oil

2 tbsp sesame seeds

2 tbsp flax seeds

½ hot pepper, thinly sliced

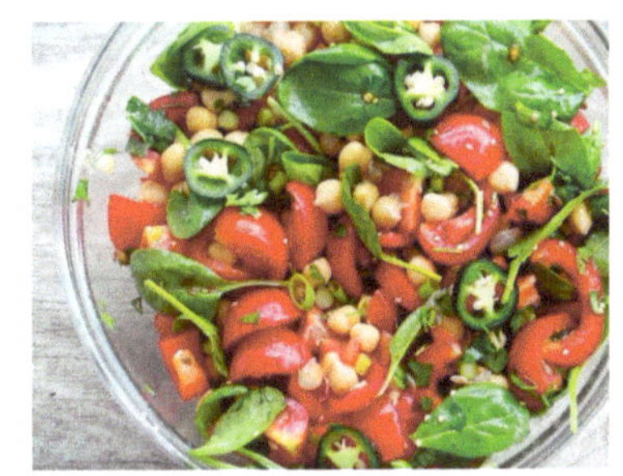

Procedure:

1. In a big mixing bowl, toss chickpeas, spinach, tomatoes, onions, pepper, and parsley.

2. Sprinkle sesame seeds and flax seeds. Mix in the rest of the vegetables.

3. Add olive oil, lemon juice, balsamic vinegar, and mix everything well.

4. Add salt to taste.

Mediterranean Chickpeas Salad in Herb Citrus Vinaigrette

Servings: 2

Preparation Time: 10 minutes

Ingredients:

Herb Citrus Vinaigrette:

2 tbsp orange juice (plus zest from ½ orange)

1 tbsp lemon juice (plus zest of ½ lemon)

1 tbsp fresh oregano, chopped

Salt, a pinch

2 tbsp olive oil

2-3 tbsp mint, julienned

Black pepper to taste

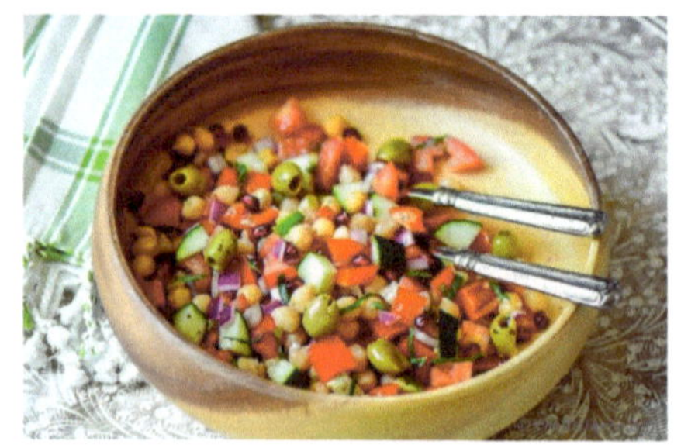

Salad:

2 cups chickpeas, cooked

1 red bell pepper, diced

½ cup red onion, diced

1 cucumber, diced

2 tomatoes, diced

¼ cup green olives

½ cup pomegranate

Procedure:

1. In a wide salad bowl, add all the ingredients on the herb citrus dressing and whisk to emulsify the oil and citrus. Season with salt and pepper and set aside.

2. Drain chickpeas and add to salad bowl with dressing.

3. Add chopped onion. Mix then set aside to let chickpeas and onion marinate in dressing.

4. Add the rest of the veggies to the salad bowl and toss to coat. Adjust seasoning.

5. Serve chilled.

Asian Salad with Peanut Dressing

Servings: 4

Prep Time: 10 minutes   Cook Time: 20 minutes

Ingredients:

Peanut salad dressing:

¼ cup rice wine vinegar

1 tsp fresh ginger, chopped, or ½ tsp ginger powder

2 tbsp Tamari soy sauce or any gluten free version

1 tbsp honey

3 tbsps sesame oil

¼ cup vegetable oil

3 tbsp creamy peanut butter

2 tbsp sesame seeds, toasted

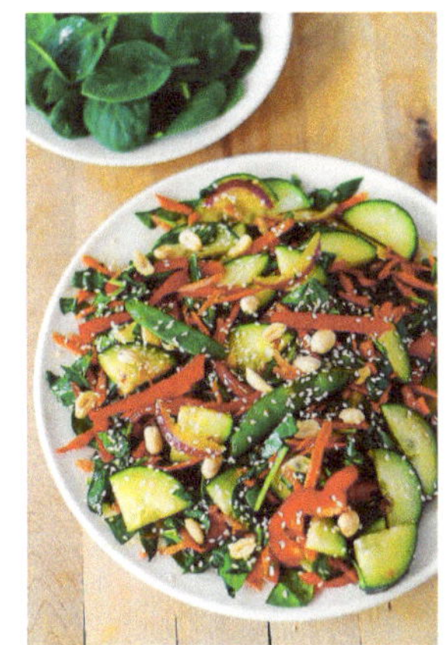

Salad:

6 cups baby spinach, wash and dried

1 carrot, shredded

1 red bell pepper, thinly sliced

¼ red onion, thinly sliced

½ pound snap peas

1 cucumber, thinly sliced

½ cup roasted peanuts

1 tbsp roasted sesame seeds

Procedure:

1. In a bowl combine all ingredients for the dressing except for 1 tbsp sesame seeds. Whisk until well combined.

2. Bring a pot of water to boil, put in the snap peas, and cook for about 5 minutes until tender.

3. Drain and rinse under very cold water. Set aside.

4. Combine all salad ingredients in one bowl. Pour the dressing over the salad, just enough to coat.

5. Sprinkle the salad with the remaining tablespoon of sesame seeds.

Power Bowls

Lentil Spaghetti Squash Power Bowl

Servings: 2

Prep Time: 10 minutes   Cook Time: 20 minutes

Ingredients:

⅓ cup lentils

1⅓ cup water

1 small roasted spaghetti squash

1 medium sweet potato, spiralized or diced,
and cooked

1 small avocado

¼ cup feta cheese

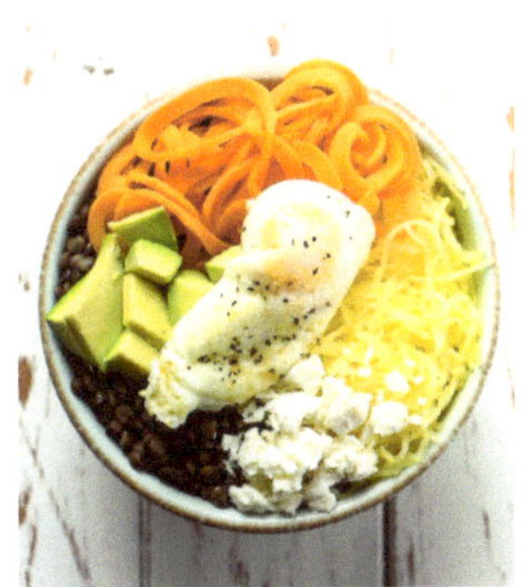

Procedure:

1. Cook the lentils: Rinse lentils in fine mesh strainer. Place in a small pot with 1⅓ cups of water and bring to a boil.

2. Reduce heat to low and simmer until tender. Remove from heat and drain water.

3. Add the lentils to your spaghetti squash as desired. Add the sweet potato, avocado, and feta.

Coconut Banana Berry Breakfast Bowl

Servings: 2

Preparation Time: 10 minutes

Ingredients:

2 cup strawberries, sliced

2 bananas, sliced

1 small handful of hemp seeds

¼ cup shredded coconut

2 tbsp cacao nibs

¼ cup chopped walnuts

2 tbsp nut butter (peanut, cashew, or almond nut butter)

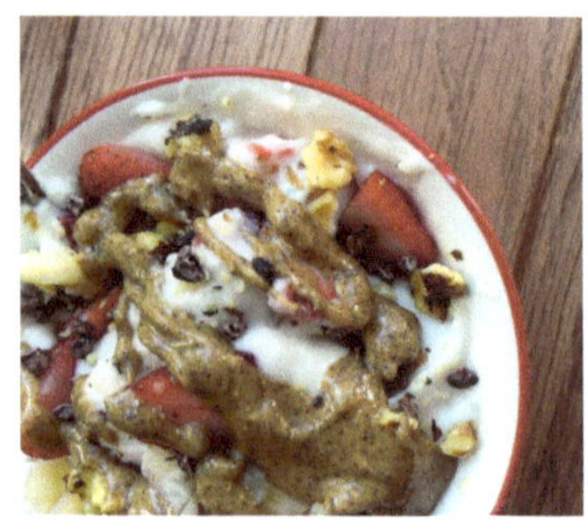

Procedure:

1. Arrange all the ingredients in a bowl.

2. A drizzle of the nut butter.

3. Serve chilled.

One Pot Mexican Quinoa

Servings: 2

Prep Time: 10 minutes   Cook Time: 20 minutes

Ingredients:

2 cloves garlic, minced

1 jalapeno, sliced

1 cup uncooked quinoa, rinsed

1 cup chicken or vegetable stock

1 can black beans, drained and rinsed

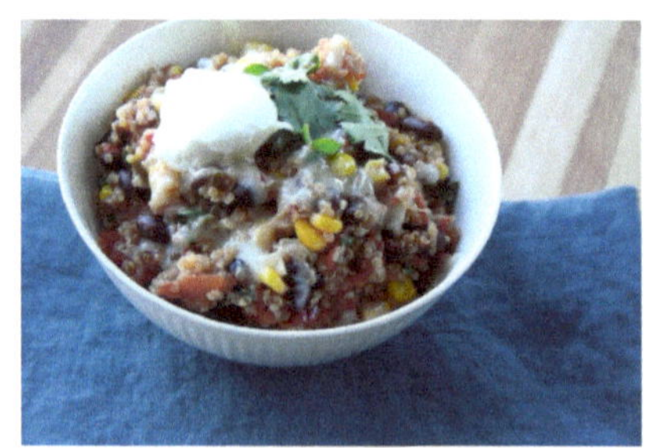

1 cup corn

1 can diced tomatoes

½ tsp salt

Juice of ¼ lime

¼ cup cilantro, chopped

Procedure:

1. In a medium pot, heat a little oil and add garlic and jalapenos, cooking until just fragrant, about 1 minute.

2. Add the quinoa, stock, beans, corn, tomatoes, and salt. Bring to a boil.

3. Lower the heat and simmer until the liquid is absorbed, about 20 minutes.

4. Stir in the lime juice and cilantro. Place in a bowl and serve.

Sushi Burrito Bowls

Servings: 2

Prep Time: 10 minutes   Cook Time: 15 minutes

Ingredients:

1 sweet potato, diced

1 tbsp olive oil

Salt and pepper

1-2 large carrots, peeled

½ - 1 cup jasmine rice, cooked

½ cup edamame

½ English cucumber, diced

1 avocado, sliced

Roasted seaweed for serving

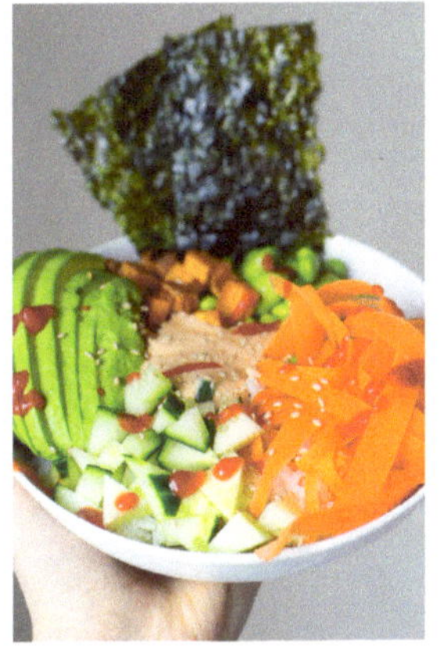

Procedure:

1. Preheat oven to 425F. Place diced sweet potatoes on a baking sheet. Add olive oil and salt and pepper to taste, and mix to combine.

2. Place in the oven for 10-15 minutes, or until potatoes are tender.

3. While the sweet potato is cooking, use a vegetable peeler to make carrot strands. Set aside.

4. When the sweet potato is tender, arrange your bowls. Divide rice between two bowls. Top with sweet potato, edamame, cucumber, avocado, roasted seaweed, and sesame seeds.

Thai Zucchini Bowls

Servings: 2

Prep Time: 10 minutes   Cook Time: 5 minutes

Ingredients:

2 ounces gluten-free pasta, cooked

2 zucchinis, spiralized

3 ½ tsp low sodium Tamari or liquid aminos

¼ cup nut butter of choice

1 ¼ tsp pressed garlic

1 ½ tsp freshly grated ginger

1 tsp Sriracha

1 tsp honey or maple syrup

Hot water, as needed

1 tbsp olive oil

2 bell peppers, sliced thinly

8 ounces mushrooms, sliced

Salt and pepper

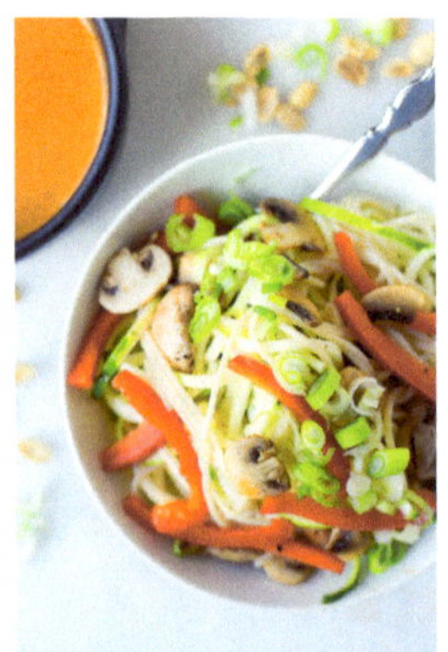

Procedure:

1. Make the sauce by adding nut butter, garlic, ginger, Sriracha, honey, and Tamari. Slowly add some water to thin and set aside.

2. In a pan over medium heat, heat olive oil and add pepper and mushroom. Cook until tender.

3. To assemble: mix pasta and zucchini in a bowl. Toss with the sauce. Top with cooked vegetables. Serve.

Asian Quinoa Power Bowl

Servings: 2

Preparation Time: 10 minutes

Ingredients:

2 cups quinoa, cooked

2 tbsp coconut oil

1 cup baby spinach

½ cup carrots, grated

½ cup edamame, shelled

¼ cup dried cranberries

2 tbsp scallions, sliced thinly

2 tbsp sesame seeds

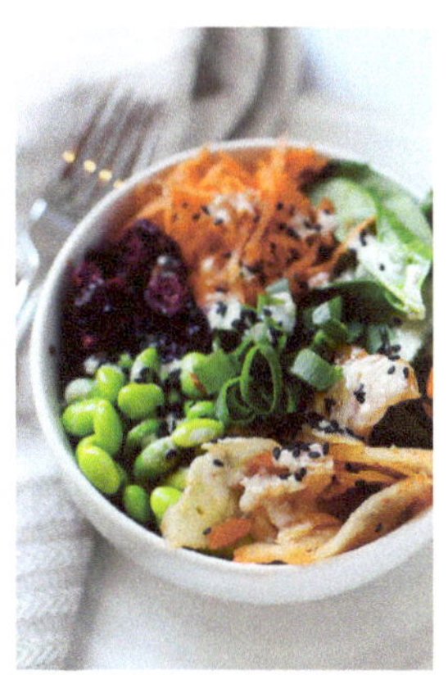

Dressing:

2 tbsp fresh ginger, grated

1 garlic clove, minced

2 tbsp white miso

2 tbsp toasted sesame oil

3 tbsp tahini

1 tbsp honey

2 tbsp lemon juice

½ cup water

Procedure:

1. To make dressing, blend all the ingredients in a blender until smooth.

2. Place cooked quinoa in bowls. Add coconut oil, and top with spinach, carrots, edamame, dried cranberries, and scallions.

3. Top with the dressing and serve.

Hawaiian Tofu BBQ Bowl

Servings: 4

Prep Time: 10 minutes   Cook Time: 20 minutes

Ingredients:

14 ounces extra firm tofu

2/3 cup uncooked quinoa

½ cup vegan barbeque sauce

Oil for cooking

Bell peppers, thinly sliced

Zucchini, thinly sliced

½ red onion, thinly sliced

½ pineapple, cored and sliced

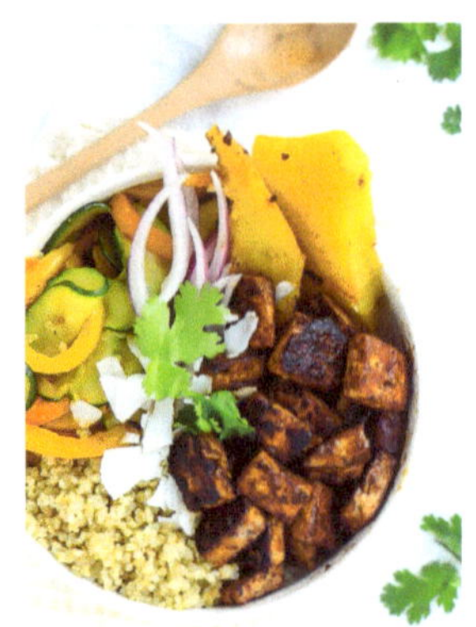

Procedure:

1. Drain the tofu, and wrap them in paper towels.

2. Heat a small saucepan over medium heat and cook the quinoa. Cook until fluffy.

3. Slice the tofu into chunks and marinate in vegan barbeque sauce.

4. In a skillet over medium heat, add oil and cook the tofu. Add bell peppers and zucchini.

5. To assemble, place quinoa in bowls and top with the tofu, veggies, onion and pineapple.

BBQ Beet Power Bowl

Servings: 2

Prep Time: 10 minutes

Ingredients:

1 cup spinach

1 small zucchini, spiralized

1 carrot, spiralized

½ cup roasted sweet potato wedges

½ cup roasted eggplant

½ cup roasted brussel sprouts

½ cup roasted beets

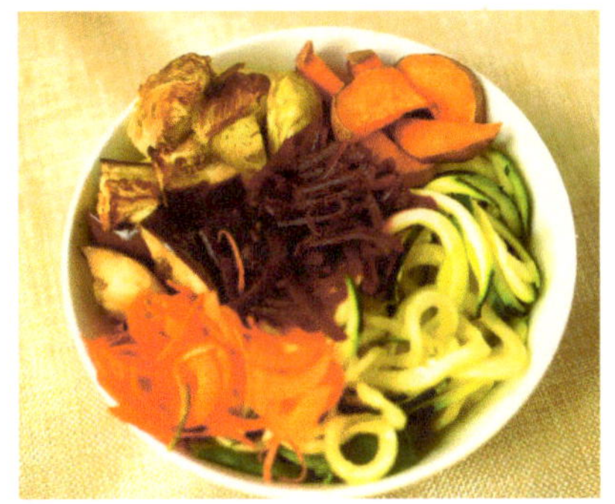

Vinaigrette:

½ cup beet juice

2 tbsp apple cider

1 tbsp olive oil

Procedure:

1.   Combine all ingredients for the vinaigrette.

2.   Assemble the rest of the ingredients in a bowl.

3.   Top with the dressing.

Macro Power Bowl

Servings: 2

Prep Time: 10 minutes

Ingredients:

1 cup cooked brown rice

1 ripe avocado, sliced

1/3 cups carrots, grated

4 radishes, sliced

½ cup snap peas, raw or steamed

½ cup fava beans, cooked

½ cup beets

Lemon and olive oil or tahini dressing

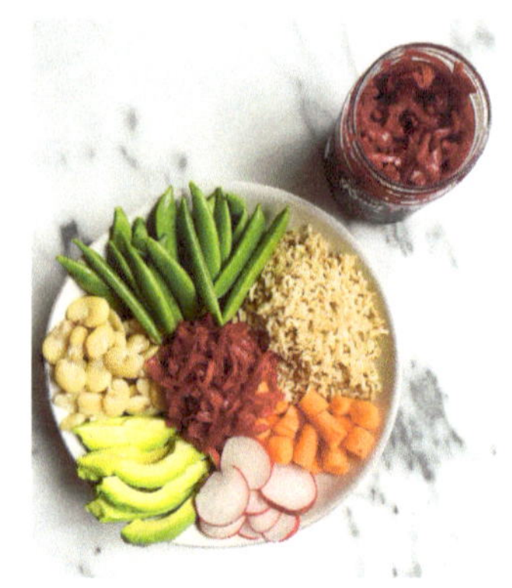

Procedure:

1. Place ingredients in a bowl.

2. Drizzle with lemon and olive oil, or tahini dressing.

Coconut Rice and Watermelon Bowl

Servings: 2

Prep Time: 10 minutes   Cook Time: 15 minutes

Ingredients:

1 cup jasmine rice

1 cup watermelon, chopped

½ cup coconut cream

1/3 cup raisins or dried blueberries

½ cup chopped basil or mint

¼ cup honey

Coconut oil

Dash of salt

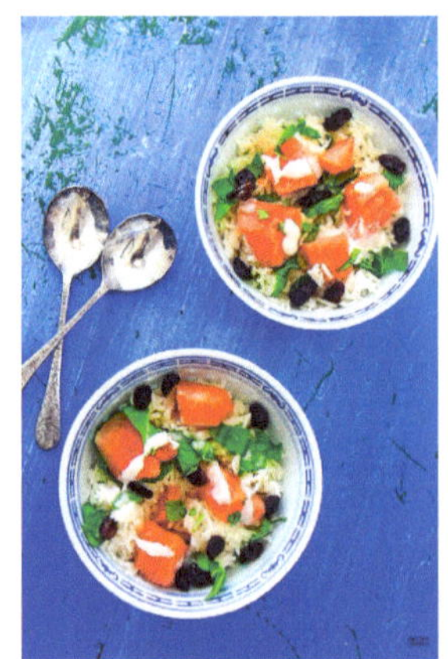

Procedure:

1. Cook rice according to package directions. Stir in 1 tbsp coconut oil and salt. Let cool once done.

2. Once cooled, add in coconut cream and honey.

3. Spoon rice into bowls and top with raisins and the rest of the toppings. Serve chilled.

Pastas

One Pan Pasta Primavera

Servings: 5

Prep Time: 10 minutes   Cook Time: 20 minutes

Ingredients:

4 tbsp olive oil

1 onion, thinly sliced

1 garlic clove, thinly sliced

350g thin spaghetti

4 cups vegetable stock

1.4g diced tomatoes with juice

140g broccoli florets

1 carrot, thinly sliced

1 tsp sea salt

140g baby spinach

70g peas

½ tsp pepper

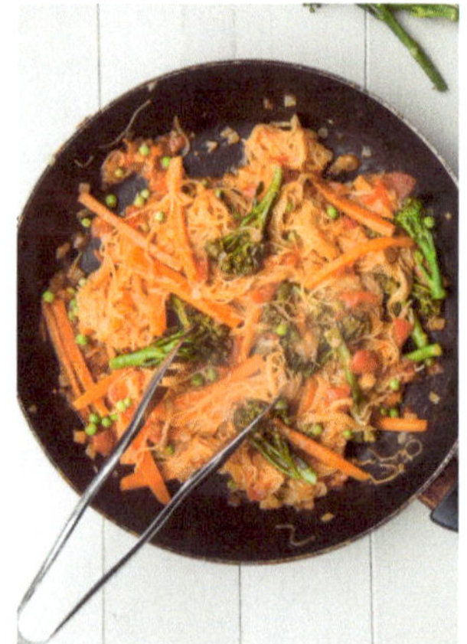

Procedure:

1.   In a pan, heat olive oil. Saute onion until soft.

2.   Add in garlic, spaghetti, vegetable stock, tomatoes, broccoli, salt, and pepper. Bring to a boil and cook until pasta is soft and liquid is absorbed.

3.   Stir in baby spinach, peas and black pepper. Toss and serve immediately.

Vegan Pot Pasta

Servings: 2

Prep Time: 10 minutes   Cook Time: 10 minutes

Ingredients:

¼ cup water

1 small onion, diced

3 garlic cloves, minced

260g mushrooms, chopped

15 g parsley, chopped

1 tsp dried oregano

1 tsp dried basil

1 tsp red pepper flakes

300 g tomatoes, diced

226 g whole wheat spiral pasta

2 cups vegetable broth

12ml coconut milk

105g chard, chopped

Salt and pepper

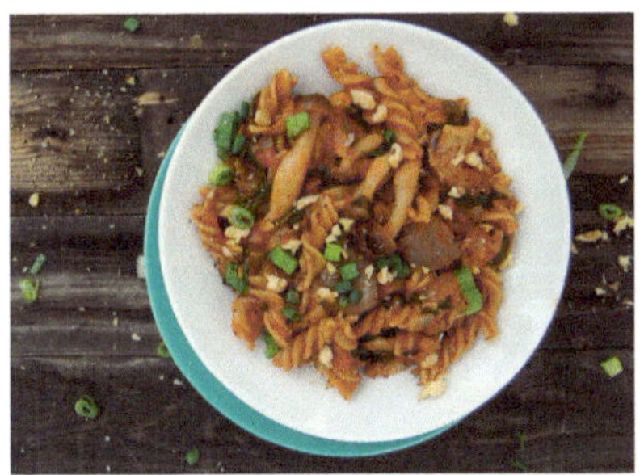

Procedure:

1. In a pan over medium heat, saute the onions and garlic.

2. Add in mushrooms, parsley, oregano, basil, garlic powder, red pepper flakes, and tomatoes.

3. Add in the pasta and vegetable broth. Bring to a boil.

4. Once pasta is done, turn off heat and add in coconut milk and chard.

5. Adjust seasoning and toss until everything is combined.

Garlic and White Wine Pasta with Brussels Sprouts

Servings: 4

Prep Time: 10 minutes   Cook Time: 20 minutes

Ingredients:

16 ounces Brussels sprouts

1-2 tbsp olive oil

1 pinch sea salt and black pepper

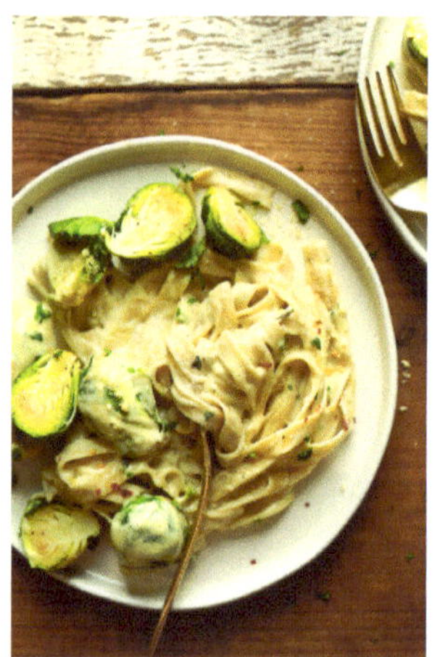

3 tbsp olive oil

4 cloves garlic, chopped

1/3 cup dry white wine

4 tbsp arrowroot

1 ¾ cup unsweetened almond milk

4 tbsp nutritional yeast

Sea salt and pepper to taste

10 ounce vegan, gluten-free pasta, cooked

Procedure:

1. Preheat oven to 400F. Place brussel sprouts on a baking sheet and drizzle with oil. Put inside oven and roast until brown on top.

2. Cook pasta until done. Set aside.

3. In a pan over medium heat, saute oil and garlic.

4. Add in wine and saute until reduced to half.

5. Whisk in arrowroot and almond milk. Transfer this to a blender and add in nutritional yeast, salt, and pepper. Blend until smooth.

6. Transfer sauce back to pan and heat until thickened.

7. Add in the brussel sprouts.

8. Toss in cooked pasta. Season accordingly.

Rainbow Thai Basil

Servings: 6

Prep Time: 15 minutes   Cook Time: 5 minutes

Ingredients:

1/3 cup Tahini

2 tbsp honey

Juice and zest of 1 lime

2 tbsp fish sauce

1 clove garlic, minced

1 tbsp ginger, grated

8 ounces rice noodles

4 cups baby kale, finely chopped

16 ounces shelled edamame

3 carrots, chopped

2 bell pepper,s sliced thinly

1 cup mango, chopped

2 stalks lemongrass, finely chopped

4 green onions, chopped

¾ cups fresh basil and cilantro

Sliced fresh peppers and roasted cashews for topping

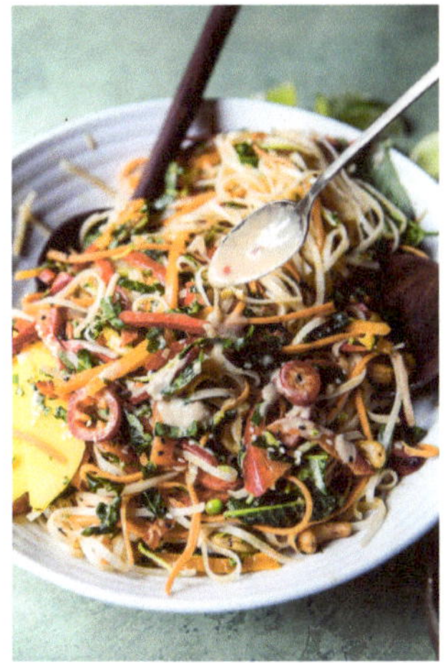

Procedure:

1. To make a vinaigrette, mix tahini, honey, lime juice and zest, fish sauce, garlic, and ginger in a mason jar. Seal the jar and shake vigorously.

2. Cook the rice noodle according to package directions. Drain and rinse.

3. Toss noodles with baby kale, edamame, carrots, bell peppers, lemongrass, green onions, herbs, and sesame seeds.

4. Drizzle with the vinaigrette and toss well to combine. Serve warm or cold.

Pesto Pasta with Artichokes and Asparagus

Servings: 6

Prep Time: 15 minutes   Cook Time: 15 minutes

Ingredients:

1 bunch asparagus

¼ cup mint leaves

⅓ cup cilantro

½ cup basil

⅓ cup pistachios

1 clove garlic, grated

Juice of 1 lemon

⅓ cup olive oil

Salt and pepper

500g long or short pasta, cooked

2 oz feta cheese

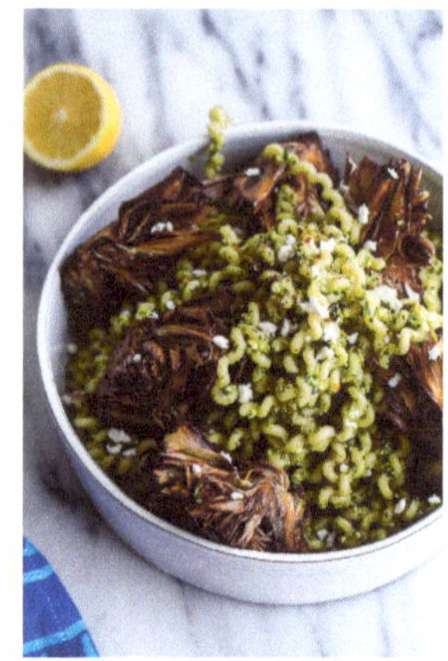

4 large artichokes

1 lemon, cut into halves

¼ cup canola oil

1 tsp lemon zest

½ tsp crushed red pepper

Sea salt

Procedure:

1.   Fill a pot with water and bring to a boil. Blanche the asparagus until tender.

2.   Put asparagus in a blender. Add mint, cilantro, basil, pistachios, garlic, lemon juice, olive oil, and salt and pulse until blended.

3. Trim the outside leaves of the artichokes. Cut into quarters and rub with lemon half.

4. Blanche the artichokes until tender and set aside.

5. In a pan over heat, fry the artichokes until crisp on all sides.

6. Toss artichokes with cilantro, lemon zest, salt, and pepper.

7. Add pesto into the cooked pasta and serve with artichokes.

Burgers and Sandwiches

Spicy Feta Chickpeas Burger

Servings: 4-6

Prep Time: 10 minutes   Cook Time: 15 minutes

Ingredients:

2 cups chickpeas, cooked

1 egg

2 tbsp olive oil

¾ cup breadcrumbs

4 tbsp cilantro

¼ cup milk

1 garlic clove, minced

¼ cup red onion, chopped

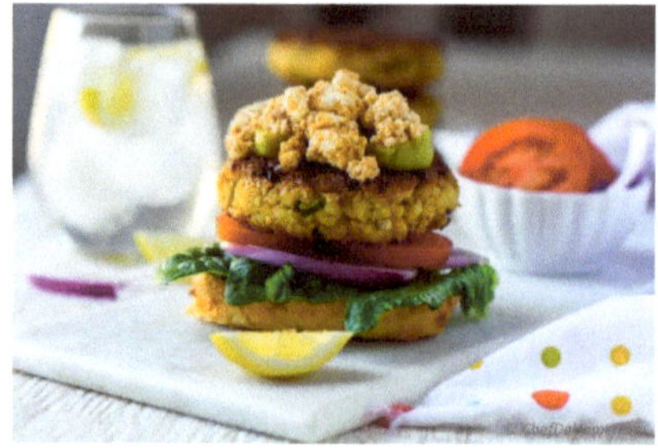

1 tbsp jalapeno, minced

1 tsp paprika

½ tsp chili flakes

½ cup feta cheese

1 tsp cumin powder

½ tsp oregano

¼ cup canola oil

4 - 6 buns

Tahini sauce

Lettuce, tomatoes (sliced)

Procedure:

1. Set aside 2 tbsp feta cheese. Heat 1 tbsp oil in a pan, add all paprika and ½ tsp cumin and remove from heat. Pour oil over remaining feta and mix well. Set aside.

2. In a large bowl, add egg, oil, salt, milk, and beat with a fork until well combined.

3. Pulse the chickpeas until coarsely chopped. Transfer into bowl with egg mixture, minced chilies, seasonings, bread crumbs, onion, garlic, and cilantro. Mix well.

4.   Divide the mixture to make 1-inch patties. Place on parchment-lined sheet, cover and refrigerate for 30 minutes to 24 hours.

5.   When ready to cook, heat a pan with oil and cook until patties are brown on each side.

6.   Serve burgers with a layer of tahini sauce on bun, layer of lettuce, tomatoes, and feta cheese.

Hemp Cauliflower Burger

Servings: 10

Prep Time: 10 minutes   Cook Time: 20 minutes

Ingredients:

Burgers:

4 flax eggs: 4 tbsp ground flaxseeds plus ¾ cup water

1 cup carrots

1 head of cauliflower

1 can garbanzo beans, drained

2 tsp garlic cloves, minced

½ cup chives, chopped

½ cup parsley, chopped

2 cups hemp seeds

1 cup almond meal

Himalayan pink salt

To serve on gluten-free buns, or lettuce

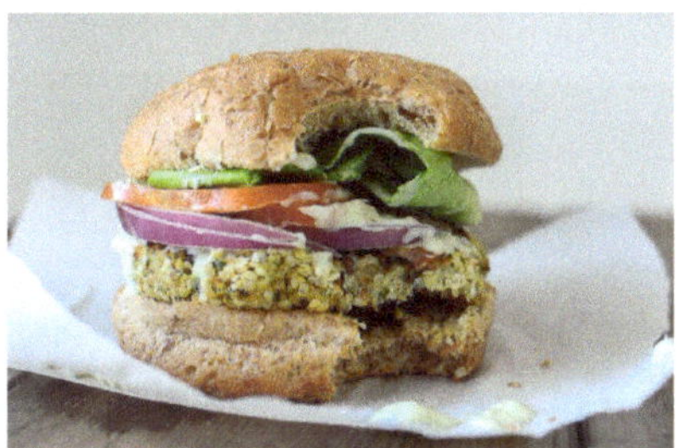

Procedure:

1.   Preheat oven to 400F.

2.   Make flax eggs by mixing 4 tbsp flaxseed with ¾ cup water in a small bowl, and set aside.

3. Wash and chop veggies. Place them on a pan line with parchment paper and bake until done.

4. Place the veggies plus garlic, chives, and parsley in a food processor and pulse until pureed but with some chunks.

5. Add hemp seeds, almond meal, flax eggs, salt and pepper to the bowl and mix well. the mixture should hold well together.

6. Shape into patties and cook in pan over medium heat.

7. Serve on lettuce over sprouted wheat and other toppings or gluten-free buns.

Sweet Potato Veggie Burgers

Servings: 6-8

Prep Time: 10 minutes   Cook Time: 20 minutes

Ingredients:

1 medium sweet potato, baked and peeled

16oz cooked white beans

½ cup white onion, diced

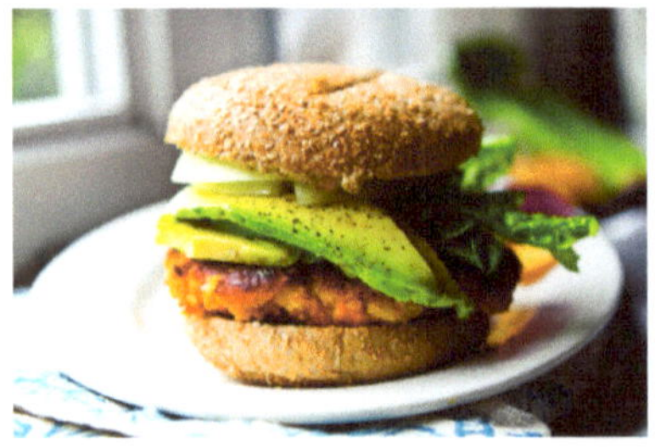

2-3 tbsp Tahini

¾ tsp Apple cider vinegar

1 tsp garlic powder

½ - 1 tsp chipotle powder

½ tsp salt

¼ tsp black pepper

1/3 cup nutritional yeast or oat flour

½ - 1 cup finely chopped greens (kale, spinach, parsley)

Panko

Toppings: avocado, tomato, vegenaise, burger buns, greens

Procedure:

1. Add the potato and beans into a bowl and mash them. Fold in onions and keep mashing.

2. Slowly add in the rest of the burger ingredients and mash until thickened.

3. Form into patties and roll them in panko to coat well.

4. In a pan over medium heat, cook both sides of the burger until browned.

5. Serve with your favorite toppings on a gluten-free or whole wheat bun.

Black Bean Plantain Burgers

Servings: 4

Prep Time: 10 minutes   Cook Time: 15 minutes

Ingredients:

1 ripe plantain, large

1 tsp virgin coconut oil

1 can black beans, drained and rinsed

¼ cup hemp seeds

1½ tbsp tahini

1 tbsp fresh lime juice

¼ cup red onion, chopped

2 tbsp cilantro, finely chopped

1-2 tbsp oat flour

¼ tsp salt + ½ tsp chipotle powder

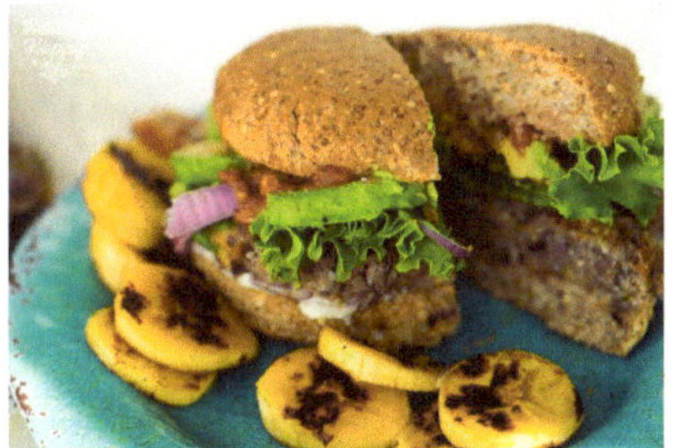

Procedure:

1. Slice plantains into rounds. Warm a skillet over heat, and add some coconut oil. Cook the round plantains until browned on all sides. Set aside 1 cup of the sliced plantains, and place them into a mixing bowl.

2. In the same mixing bowl, add black beans, chipotle powder, salt, onion, hemp seeds, tahini, lime, cilantro, and oat flour. Use a fork or potato masher, and mash well. Form into patties.

3. Warm skillet and cook the burgers until brown on both sides.

4. Assemble the cooked patties over whole wheat bun with your favorite toppings.

Mediterranean Tabouleh Burger

Servings: 10

Prep Time: 10 minutes   Cook Time: 20 minutes

Ingredients:

1 cup packed parsley leaves

½ cup mint leaves

4 scallions, chopped

1 garlic clove, chopped

1 tbsp olive oil

1½ cups cooked freekeh, cooled

1 tbsp fresh lemon juice

Sea salt and fresh ground black pepper

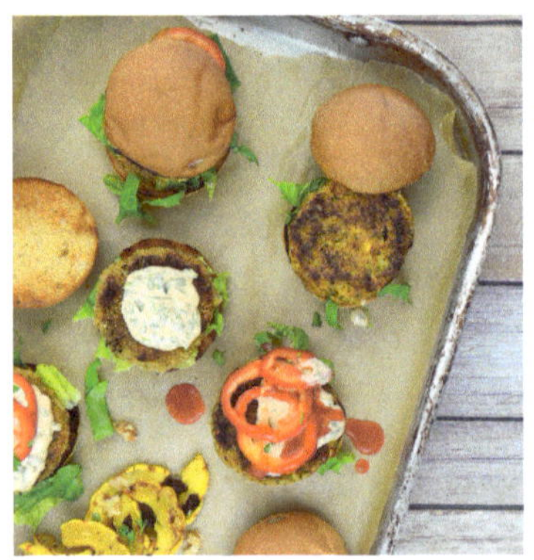

¾ cup quick cooking oatmeal

¼ cup vegetable broth

15.5oz chickpeas, rinsed and drained

1 tsp paprika

½ tsp red chili flakes

Zest of 1 lemon

10 gluten-free slider buns, toasted

Tahini-LemonSauce:

¼ cup Tahini

3 tbsp fresh lemon juice

2 tbsp water

1-2 tsp Sriracha sauce

3 tbsp finely chopped parsley

1 garlic clove, minced

Sea salt and pepper

Procedure:

1. To make the sauce, combine all ingredients in a bowl and mix well. Set aside.

2. In a food processor, combine parsley, mint, scallions, garlic, and oil in a food processor. Process until fine and transfer to a large bowl.

3. Add the freekeh, lemon juice, and season with salt and pepper.

4. Heat the oatmeal and broth in a saucepan over medium heat. Stir and cook until thickened. Transfer this to freekeh mixture.

5. Add the chickpeas, paprika, chili flakes, and lemon zest in a food processor. Pulse to break the chickpeas into smaller pieces. Transfer to the freekeh mixture.

6. Mix the burger mixture well. Adjust seasoning and form into patties.

7. In a pan over medium heat, cook the burgers until brown on both sides.

8. Assemble the burgers with your favorite gluten-free bread and toppings.

Casseroles

Mexican Style Beans and Rice Casserole

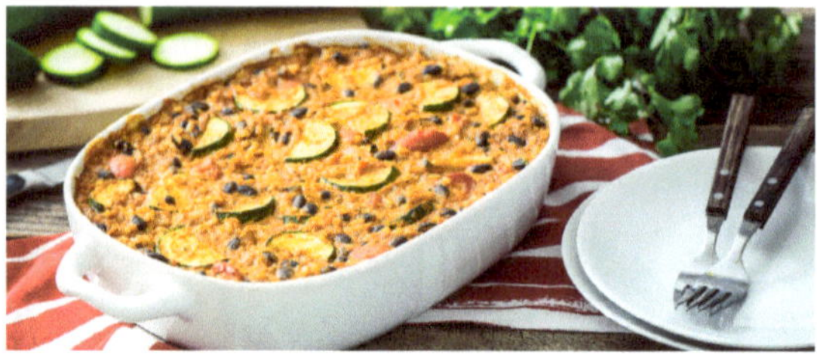

Servings: 6-8

Prep Time: 10 minutes   Cook Time: 20 minutes

Ingredients:

1 large yellow onion, diced

1 red bell pepper, diced

3 cloves garlic, minced

1 tbsp cumin seeds, toasted

2 tsps ancho chili powder

2 medium zucchini, diced

2 cups cooked brown rice

2 cups cooked black beans

3 ears corn, kernels removed

Cilantro, chopped

Procedure:

1. Preheat oven to 350F.

2. Saute onions and peppers in a large saucepan over medium heat.

3. Add water to keep them sticking to the pan. Add the garlic.

4. Add cumin and chili powder and cook for another 30 seconds.

5. Remove from heat. Add the cooked rice, zucchini, black beans, corn, and mix well.

6. Spoon the mixture into an 8x8 baking dish. Bake until bubbly. Serve with cilantro on top.

Hearty Tu-No Casserole

Servings: 6-8

Prep Time: 10 minutes   Cook Time: 20 minutes

Ingredients:

Sauce:

2½ cups almond/ soy milk

½ cup cashews

1 tsp onion, minced

½ tsp pepper

1 tbsp kelp powder

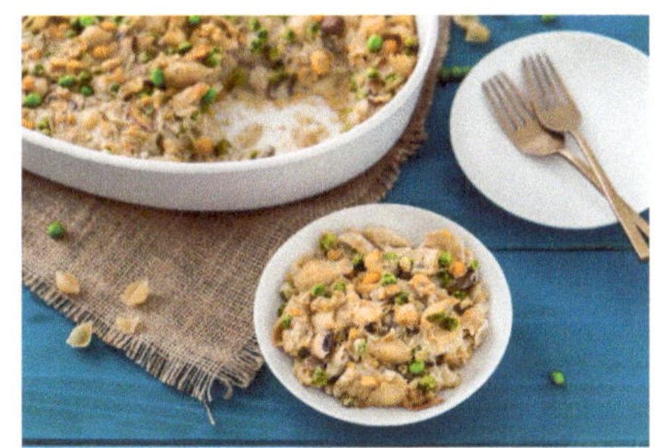

Base:

1½ cups shell pasta, cooked

1 yellow onion, chopped

8 cremini mushrooms, sliced

2 cups green peas

3 cups cooked garbanzo beans

Procedure:

1.   Preheat oven to 375F.

2.   Place the plant milk, cashews, onion, pepper, and kelp in a blender and blend until smooth.

3.   Add the onions and mushrooms to a skillet over high heat and saute until tender. Add this along with the peas to the cooked pasta. Mix in the mixture from step 2.

4.   Pulse garbanzo beans in a food processor until smooth. Add this to the pasta mixture.

5.   Spoon the mixture to a baking dish and cook in oven until top is lightly browned.

Shepherd's Pot Pie

Servings: 6-8

Prep Time: 10 minutes   Cook Time: 20 minutes

Ingredients:

4 large russet potatoes, boiled, mashed and seasoned with sea salt and pepper

2 large yellow onions, finely diced

3 large carrots, diced

3 cups frozen peas

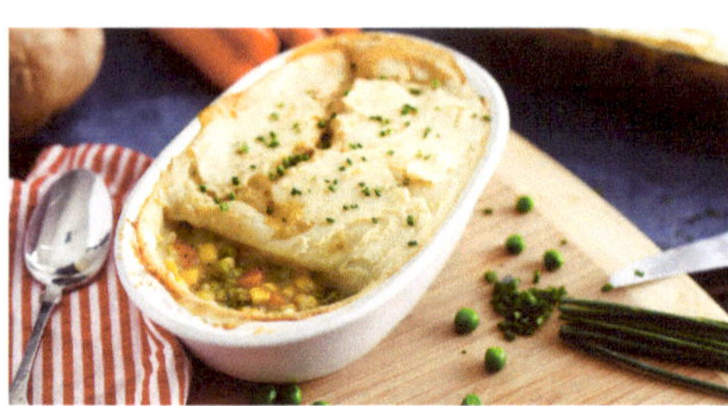

3 cups frozen corn

4 cups frozen broccoli florets

6 tbsp arrowroot powder

4 cups unsweetened, unflavored plant milk

¼ cup nutritional yeast

freshly ground black pepper

Chives, chopped

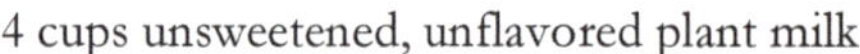

Procedure:

1. Preheat oven to 350F.

2. Saute onions and carrots in a pan until tender.

3. Add the peas, corn, and broccoli. Cook until heated through.

4. Combine the arrowroot powder with the plant milk in a bowl and whisk until blended.

5. Add this mixture to the vegetables along with the nutritional yeast. Cook until thickened.

6. Adjust seasoning. Transfer the mixture to a pan and top with mashed potatoes.

7. Bake in oven until top is slightly brown.

Tacos

Kale Tacos

Servings: 2

Prep Time: 10 minutes   Cook Time: 10 minutes

Ingredients:

1 cup black beans, cooked
1 cup kale, finely chopped
¼ clove garlic, crushed
½ avocado, sliced
8 small tacos
1 cup onions, finely chopped
1 cup tomatoes, finely chopped
2 tbsp cilantro, finely chopped
½ lemon
Salt

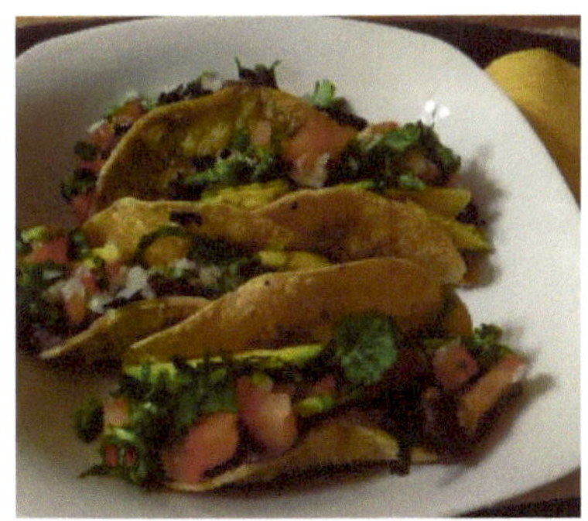

Procedure:

1. Season the black beans with salt and cumin powder and mash into a mush.
2. In a pan, cook kale and garlic together with 1 tbsp water, until soft.
3. Toast tacos on the skillet. Fold into half and stack on a plate.
4. Spread 1 tbsp of black bean sauce on one side of the taco and top with sautéed kale, avocado, onions, tomatoes, cilantro, and lemon juice.
5. Fold the taco and set aside.
6. Repeat for the rest of the tacos. Serve immediately.

Guacamole Tacos

Servings: 2

Prep Time: 8 minutes   Cook Time: 20 minutes

Ingredients:

Guacamole:

2 avocados, pit and skin removed

½ lime

½ lemon

¼ tsp salt

⅓ cup corn kernels

¼ cup red belle pepper, diced

2 tbsp diced Poblano pepper, diced

1 tbsp red onion, diced

1 tbsp jalapeno pepper, diced

2 tsp cilantro, minced

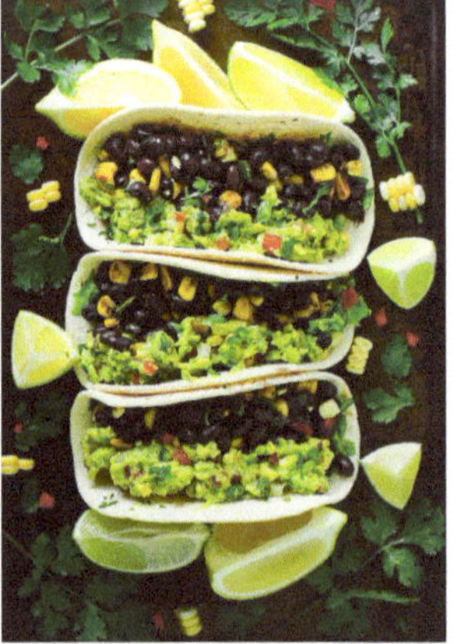

Beans:

15 ounces black beans

1/3 cup corn kernels

¼ cup red bell pepper, diced

¼ cup poblano peppers, diced

½ tsp ground cumin

Tacos:

6 small flour or corn tortillas

2 cups chopped iceberg or romaine lettuce

1 tbsp cilantro, minced

Lime wedges

Procedure:

1. To make guacamole: mash the avocado in a bowl with a fork. Add a squeeze of lime and lemon. Add salt. Add in the rest of guacamole ingredients and set aside.
2. Add all the ingredients for the black beans in a pot and heat until soft.
3. Line each tortilla with lettuce, spoon the black bean mixture over. Spoon the guacamole.
4. Top with cilantro and serve with some lime wedges.

Vegan Mushroom Tacos

Servings: 4

Prep Time: 15 minutes   Cook Time: 15 minutes

Ingredients:

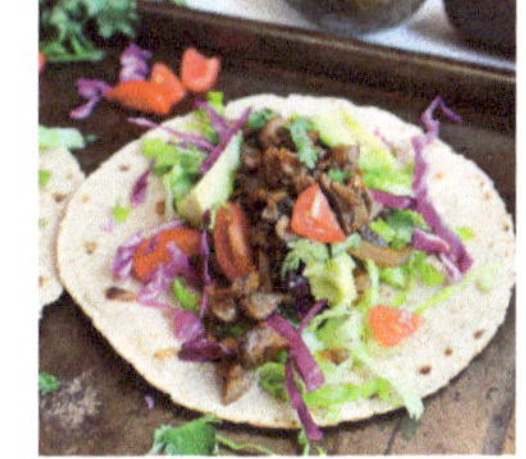

8 ounces mushrooms, diced

1 onion, diced

½ red bell pepper, diced

1 tbsp balsamic vinegar

1 tsp cocoa powder

1 tsp smoked paprika

1 tsp Braggs aminos

1 pack tortilla shells

Procedure:

1. Add a few tablespoons of water to a pan over heat.
2. Saute onions and bell pepper in the water until translucent.
3. Add mushrooms and remaining ingredients and cook until done.
4. Build tacos by placing the filling inside with your favorite toppings.

Falafel Tacos

Servings: 5

Prep Time: 10 minutes   Cook Time: 10 minutes

Ingredients:

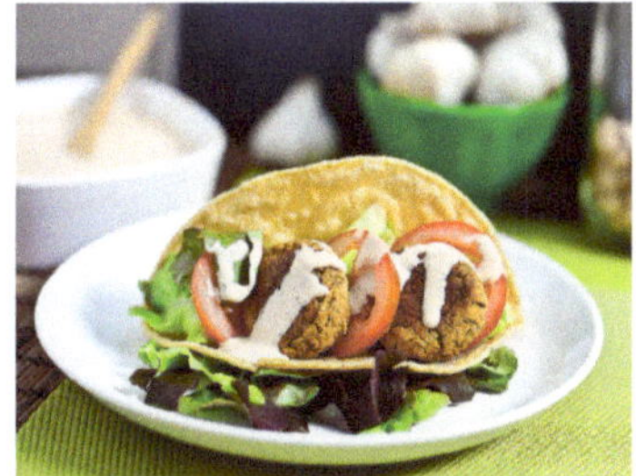

10 corn tortillas

10-12 baked falafel

1 cup of your favorite salsa

2 cups romaine, chopped

1 large tomato, chopped

1 medium red onion, chopped

Procedure:

1. Heat a non-stick pan over medium heat. Add corn tortillas to cover the bottom of the pan. Soften the tortillas and repeat with the other tortillas.
2. To serve, cut each falafel in half, and place two or three halves in the center of each tortilla.
3. Top with salsa, romaine, tomatoes, and red onions.

Orange Black Bean Taquitos

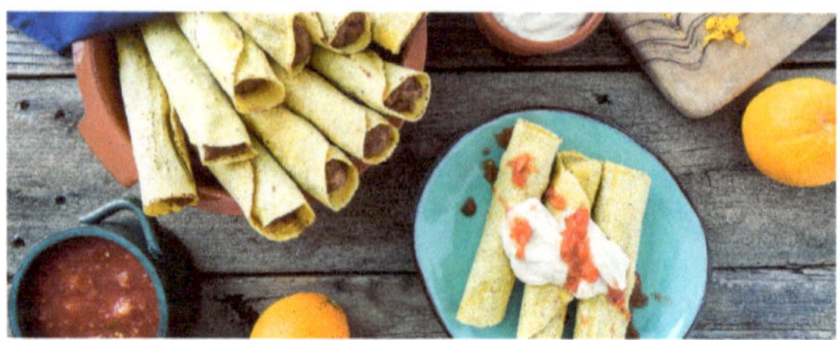

Servings: 5

Prep Time: 10 minutes   Cook Time: 10 minutes

Ingredients:

1 large yellow onion, diced

4 cloves garlic, minced

2 tsp cumin seeds, toasted and grounded

2 tsp ancho powder

Zest and juice of 2 oranges

15 ounces black beans, drained and rinsed

Sea salt

10 corn tortillas

Salsa of choice

Procedure:

1. Saute the onions and garlic until translucent. Add the cumin, ancho powder, orange zest, and juice.
2. Add in the black beans, and season with salt to taste.
3. Transfer to a food processor and pulse until smooth but a still a bit chunky.
4. Place the tortillas over a hot skillet until softened.
5. Spread 3 tbsp of the black bean mixture over half of the tortilla. Roll it up and do the same for the rest.
6. Serve with salsa of choice.

Conclusion

The whole-foods plant-based diet is a wonderful way of letting you experience a whole new reality of healthy living. This book was written to provide you with more Lunch and Dinner recipes so that you will continue to feel better, healthier, happier, and have more vitality for life than you ever did before.

To find out more about the whole foods plant-based diet, as well as recipes for breakfast, lunch and dinner, dessert and beverages, do get a copy of the *Whole Foods Plant-based Cookbook With Recipes In 30 Minutes*.

I wish you all the health, happiness, and love you deserve in life.

-- Esther Keller

www.ingramcontent.com/pod-product-compliance
Lightning Source LLC
Chambersburg PA
CBHW040308240726
48664CB00006B/1420